The Ultimate Guide to Castor Oil: Unleashing the

Power of Nature's Elixir

Introduction:

1. Welcome to the World of Castor Oil

   - Brief history and origins

   - Overview of castor oil extraction process

   - Importance and versatility of castor oil

Chapter 1: Castor Oil Basics

1. What is Castor Oil?

   - Introduction to castor oil composition and properties

   - Differentiating between cold-pressed and refined castor oil

2. The Science Behind Castor Oil

   - Chemical composition and beneficial compounds

   - Understanding the unique structure of ricinoleic acid

3. How is Castor Oil Produced?

   - Insights into the castor bean plant and cultivation

   - Detailed extraction methods and production techniques

Chapter 2: Health and Beauty Applications

1. Castor Oil for Skin Care

   - Nourishing and moisturizing properties

   - Treating common skin conditions (acne, dryness, etc.)

   - DIY recipes for face masks, cleansers, and more

2. Revitalizing Hair with Castor Oil

   - Promoting hair growth and preventing hair loss

- A glossary of key terms related to castor oil and its applications.

Introduction

Welcome to the enchanting world of castor oil, where nature's elixir holds a wealth of secrets waiting to be discovered. In this comprehensive guide, "The Ultimate Guide to Castor Oil: Unleashing the Power of Nature's Elixir," we invite you to embark on a transformative journey that will unravel the mysteries and unveil the remarkable properties of castor oil. Throughout history, castor oil has been revered for its diverse range of applications and its ability to provide natural remedies and solutions. From ancient civilizations to modern times, this extraordinary oil has captivated the attention of herbalists, healers, and beauty enthusiasts alike. Its origins can be traced back to the castor bean plant, a remarkable botanical wonder that continues to flourish across the globe.

Within the pages of this guide, we will embark on a captivating exploration of castor oil's history, extraction methods, and its significance in various industries. We will dive into the science behind castor oil, unraveling its chemical composition and unique properties that make it a powerhouse of natural goodness. Whether you are a curious beginner or a seasoned enthusiast, this guide will equip you with the knowledge you need to harness the full potential of castor oil.

In the chapters that follow, we will delve into the captivating world of castor oil applications. We will unveil its beauty secrets, from nourishing and rejuvenating the skin to revitalizing hair and enhancing nail health. Discover how castor oil can be your trusted ally on the journey to radiant beauty.

But castor oil's benefits extend far beyond beauty. We will explore its remarkable healing properties, from soothing digestive discomfort to relieving joint and muscle pain. Discover the immune-boosting potential of castor oil and its role in detoxification and cleansing.

Castor oil's versatility is not limited to personal care and wellness. We will uncover its presence in the industrial realm, where it finds applications in lubricants and various manufacturing processes. From cosmetics to household products, castor oil plays an essential role in countless everyday items.

As you navigate through this guide, we will provide safety guidelines and precautions to ensure your experience with castor oil is both enjoyable and beneficial. Learn how to choose high-quality castor oil and understand the proper storage methods to preserve its potency.

So, whether you seek a natural remedy, a beauty enhancer, or a sustainable solution, castor oil has something extraordinary to offer. Join us as we embark on a journey to unlock the boundless potential of nature's elixir. Prepare to be inspired, informed, and empowered to embrace the remarkable benefits of castor oil in your daily life. Let us begin this transformative adventure together.

Chapter 1: Castor Oil Basics

What is Castor Oil?

Castor oil, derived from the seeds of the castor bean plant (Ricinus communis), is a versatile vegetable oil with a long history of use. Castor oil is known for its pale yellow to amber color and distinct, earthy aroma.

It is composed primarily of triglycerides, with ricinoleic acid being the dominant fatty acid, accounting for its unique properties.

The Science Behind Castor Oil

Ricinoleic acid: Castor oil's key component, ricinoleic acid, is a monounsaturated fatty acid known for its remarkable properties, including anti-inflammatory, antimicrobial, and analgesic effects.

Viscosity: Castor oil has a thick, sticky consistency due to its high viscosity, making it useful for various applications.

How is Castor Oil Produced?

Castor bean cultivation: The castor bean plant is native to tropical and subtropical regions. It thrives in well-drained soils and warm climates.

Extraction methods: Castor oil is obtained by extracting oil from castor beans. Two primary extraction methods are commonly used: cold-pressing and refining.

Cold-pressing: In this method, castor beans are mechanically pressed to extract oil without the use of heat or chemical solvents. It results in a pure, unrefined form of castor oil, often referred to as "cold-pressed castor oil."

Refining: Refined castor oil undergoes additional processing steps to remove impurities and enhance its clarity and stability. It may involve processes like degumming, bleaching, and deodorization.

Castor Oil Grades and Types

Different grades: Castor oil is available in various grades, including pharmaceutical grade, industrial grade, and cosmetic grade, depending on its intended use and level of purity.

Organic and conventional: Castor oil can be produced organically, following strict organic farming practices, or conventionally, using standard agricultural methods.

Understanding the basics of castor oil sets the foundation for exploring its wide-ranging applications. In the upcoming chapters, we will delve deeper into the remarkable uses of casto oil for health, beauty, wellness, and industrial purposes. By harnessing the power of this natural elixir, you can unlock a world of possibilities. Let's embark on an exciting journey to unleash the potential of castor oil together.

Historical Significance

Castor oil has a rich history that spans centuries and cultures. It has been used for various purposes throughout history, from ancient Egypt and Greece to traditional Ayurvedic and Chinese medicine. In ancient Egypt, castor oil was highly regarded for its healing properties and was even found in ancient tombs. It was used in skincare, haircare, and as a natural remedy for ailments. Traditional Ayurvedic medicine considers castor oil to be a potent detoxifying agent and has used it for cleansing and promoting overall well-being. Castor oil has also found its place in traditional Chinese medicine, where it is believed to invigorate blood circulation and alleviate pain.

Global Production and Trade

- Castor oil is produced in several countries worldwide, with India, China, and Brazil being the largest producers.

- India has a long-standing history of castor oil production and is known for its quality castor beans and extraction techniques.

- The global trade of castor oil is significant, with various industries relying on its unique properties for their products.

Sustainability and Eco-friendliness

- Castor oil holds ecological advantages, as the castor bean plant is highly resilient and requires minimal pesticides or fertilizers.

- The plant's byproducts, such as castor meal and castor pomace, can be repurposed for organic fertilizers or used in industrial applications.

- Castor oil is considered a renewable resource, making it an eco-friendly choice compared to petroleum-based alternatives.

Unique Properties of Castor Oil

Hydration and Moisturization: Castor oil is renowned for its exceptional moisturizing properties. Its high viscosity forms a protective barrier on the skin, helping to retain moisture and prevent dryness.

Anti-inflammatory Effects: Ricinoleic acid, the primary component of castor oil, exhibits potent anti-inflammatory properties. It can help soothe and calm irritated skin, making it beneficial for conditions like eczema, dermatitis, and sunburn.

Hair Nourishment and Growth: Castor oil has been used for centuries to promote hair growth and enhance hair health. It helps nourish the hair follicles, strengthens the hair shaft, and may even address issues like hair loss and thinning.

Antimicrobial Activity: Castor oil possesses antimicrobial properties, making it effective against certain bacteria and fungi. It can be used to address scalp infections, fungal conditions, and even as a natural alternative to conventional antiseptics.

Traditional and Folk Remedies

Castor oil has a rich tradition in folk remedies across various cultures. It has been used to alleviate constipation, promote bowel movements, and support digestive health.

Traditional uses also include castor oil packs, where a cloth soaked in castor oil is applied to the skin to aid in detoxification, relieve pain, and support organ function.

Oral ingestion of castor oil in small amounts has been used to stimulate labor during childbirth, although this practice should only be undertaken under professional supervision.

Safety Considerations and Precautions

While castor oil is generally considered safe, some individual may be sensitive or allergic to it. It is advisable to perform a patch test before using castor oil topically or orally.

Oral consumption of castor oil should be done sparingly and under professional guidance, as excessive intake may lead to digestive discomfort or other adverse effects. It is important to choose high-quality castor oil and store it properly to maintain its freshness and efficacy.

Allergic Reactions and Sensitivities

Although rare, some individuals may have allergic reactions or sensitivities to castor oil. Before using castor oil topically, perform a patch test by applying a small amount to a small area of skin and observing for any adverse reactions such as redness, itching, or irritation.

Note: If you experience any signs of an allergic reaction, discontinue use immediately and consult a healthcare professional.

Choosing High-Quality Castor Oil

Ensure that you select high-quality, pure castor oil for optimal effectiveness and safety. Look for cold-pressed or organic castor oil options, as these tend to retain more of the natural beneficial compounds. Check for reputable brands and read product labels to ensure you are purchasing a reliable and authentic product.

Proper Storage and Shelf Life

Store castor oil in a cool, dark place away from direct sunlight to maintain its potency and extend its shelf life. Castor oil has a relatively long shelf life, usually ranging from one to two years, but it is still advisable to check the expiration date and discard any expired products.

Avoid Contact with Eyes and Mucous Membranes

Keep castor oil away from direct contact with the eyes and mucous membranes, as it can cause irritation and discomfort. If accidental contact occurs, rinse the affected area thoroughly with water and seek medical attention if necessary.

Consult a Healthcare Professional

If you have any underlying health conditions, are pregnant or breastfeeding, or are taking medications, it is advisable to consult a healthcare professional before using castor oil. They can provide personalized guidance and ensure that castor oil is safe for your specific circumstances.

Chapter 2: Health and Beauty Applications

n Chapter 2 of "The Comprehensive Guide to Castor Oil: Unleashing the Power of Nature's Elixir," we delve into the captivating realm of health and beauty applications. Castor oil's remarkable properties make it a popular choice for enhancing our well-being and nurturing our external appearance. Get ready to discover the transformative effects of castor oil in skincare, haircare, and nail health.

Castor Oil for Skin Care

Nourishing and Hydrating Properties: Castor oil's ric
consistency helps lock in moisture, providing deep hydration t
the skin. It can be used to alleviate dryness, rough patches, an
flaky skin.

Anti-Aging Benefits: The antioxidant properties of castor o
may help reduce the appearance of fine lines, wrinkles, and ag
spots. It promotes a more youthful and radiant complexion.

Soothing and Calming Effects: Castor oil's anti-inflammator
properties make it effective in soothing irritated and inflame
skin conditions, such as acne, eczema, and dermatitis.

Revitalizing Hair with Castor Oil

Stimulating Hair Growth: Castor oil is renowned for its ability to promote hair growth. It nourishes the scalp, strengthens the hair follicles, and may help address hair loss or thinning.

Conditioning and Moisturizing: Castor oil acts as an excellent natural conditioner, providing deep hydration and improving the overall texture and shine of the hair.

Taming Frizz and Split Ends: The emollient properties of castor oil help control frizz, reduce flyaways, and seal split ends, leading to smoother and more manageable hair.

Scalp Health and Dandruff Relief: Castor oil's antimicrobial and anti-inflammatory properties can assist in maintaining a healthy scalp, reducing dandruff, and soothing itchiness.

DIY Haircare Recipes: Discover simple homemade hair masks, scalp treatments, and serums that harness the power of castor oil for luscious locks.

Enhancing Nail and Cuticle Health

Strengthening Weak and Brittle Nails: Castor oil's nourishing properties can help fortify weak and brittle nails, promoting strength and resilience.

Conditioning Cuticles: Regular application of castor oil to the cuticles can moisturize and soften them, preventing dryness, hangnails, and potential infections.

Nail Growth and Health: Castor oil's ability to enhance circulation can contribute to healthier nail growth and reduce the occurrence of breakage and splitting.

Chapter 3: Healing & Wellness

Castor Oil for Digestive Health

Relieving Constipation: Castor oil is renowned for its gentle laxative properties, making it an effective natural remedy for relieving occasional constipation.

Promoting Regularity: By stimulating bowel movements, castor oil can help establish a regular digestive pattern and improve overall gut health.

Soothing Gastrointestinal Discomfort: The anti-inflammatory properties of castor oil can help reduce inflammation in the digestive tract, providing relief from discomfort and bloating.

Alleviating Joint and Muscle Pain

Anti-inflammatory Effects: Castor oil's anti-inflammatory properties can help reduce swelling and inflammation associated with joint pain, arthritis, and muscle soreness.

Joint Lubrication and Mobility: Regular application of castor oil to joints can help lubricate them, promoting smoother movement and potentially alleviating stiffness.

Castor Oil Packs: Castor oil packs, when applied topically to affected areas, can provide localized relief and relaxation, making them beneficial for muscle and joint discomfort.

Immune System Support and Detoxification

Immune-Boosting Properties: Castor oil is believed to have immune-stimulating effects, supporting the body's natural defense mechanisms and promoting overall immune system health.

Detoxification and Cleansing: Castor oil packs applied to the abdomen can help stimulate lymphatic drainage and support the body's detoxification processes, aiding in the elimination of toxins.

Supporting Skin Healing and Wound Care

Promoting Wound Healing: Castor oil's antimicrobial and anti inflammatory properties can assist in wound healing by reducing the risk of infection and supporting the skin's natural healing processes.

Soothing Skin Conditions: The soothing and moisturizing effects of castor oil make it beneficial for addressing skin conditions such as sunburns, rashes, and minor cuts or scrapes.

Scar Reduction: Regular application of castor oil to scars may help soften and minimize their appearance over time.

Supporting Menstrual Health

Castor oil has been traditionally used to promote menstrual health and alleviate menstrual discomfort. Applying castor oil packs to the lower abdomen during menstruation may help soothe cramps, reduce inflammation, and provide relief from menstrual pain. The gentle heat generated by the castor oil pack can also aid in relaxation and promote a sense of comfort during menstruation.

Addressing Fungal Infections

Castor oil possesses antifungal properties that can help combat various fungal infections, such as athlete's foot, ringworm, and fungal nail infections.

Regular application of castor oil to affected areas may help inhibit the growth of fungi and support the healing process.

Supporting Liver Health

Castor oil packs applied to the right side of the abdomen, where the liver is located, are believed to have a detoxifying effect on this vital organ. The packs can help stimulate liver function, promote bile flow, and aid in the elimination of toxins from the body.

Easing Discomfort from Hemorrhoids

Castor oil can provide relief from the discomfort associated with hemorrhoids. Applying castor oil topically to the affected area can help reduce inflammation, soothe itching, and promote healing.

Enhancing Sleep and Relaxation

The calming properties of castor oil, along with its moisturizing effects on the skin, make it an excellent addition to nighttime relaxation rituals.

A gentle massage with castor oil can promote relaxation, soothe the senses, and enhance the quality of sleep.

Chapter 4: Industrial and Household Applications

Castor Oil in Cosmetics and Personal Care Products

Cosmetic Industry Applications: Castor oil finds extensive use in the cosmetics industry due to its emollient, moisturizing, and film-forming properties. It is commonly found in lipsticks, foundations, mascaras, and various skincare formulations.

Emulsifying Agent: Castor oil acts as an emulsifying agent, helping to blend oil and water-based ingredients in cosmetic formulations, ensuring stability and uniformity.

Castor Oil in Lubricants and Industrial Uses

Lubricant Applications: Castor oil's high viscosity and lubricating properties make it ideal for use in machinery, engines, and other mechanical applications. It can help reduce friction, prevent wear and tear, and provide long-lasting lubrication.

Hydraulic Fluids: Castor oil's resistance to high temperature and its ability to maintain its viscosity under pressure make it suitable for use as hydraulic fluids in various industries.

Plastics and Resins: Castor oil derivatives are used in the production of biodegradable plastics, resins, and coatings offering a sustainable alternative to petroleum-based products.

Textiles and Leather Industry: Castor oil is used as a finishing agent in textiles and leather processing, providing softness, flexibility, and water repellency to the final products.

Household and DIY Applications

Natural Wood Polish: Castor oil can be used as a natural alternative to commercial wood polishes, providing a protective and nourishing coating to enhance the natural beauty of wooden surfaces.

Leather Conditioner: Castor oil helps condition and restore suppleness to leather items such as shoes, bags, and furniture.

Lubricating Household Tools: Applying a small amount of castor oil to hinges, locks, and other household tools can help reduce friction and ensure smooth operation.

Natural Stain Remover: Castor oil can be effective in removing stains from fabrics and upholstery. It helps break down grease and oil-based stains, making them easier to remove.

Castor Oil in Soap and Detergent Manufacturing

Castor oil is commonly used in soap and detergent formulations due to its ability to produce rich, creamy lather and its cleansing properties. It helps to remove dirt, oil, and impurities from the skin and fabrics, making it an essential ingredient in soaps shampoos, laundry detergents, and other cleansing products. Castor oil contributes to the moisturizing and conditioning effects of these products, leaving the skin and hair feeling sof and nourished.

Castor Oil in Candle Making

Castor oil is used in the production of candles, particularly in the creation of longer-lasting and drip-free candles.

It helps to increase the melting point and hardness of the candle wax, allowing for a slow and even burn with minimal smoke and soot. Castor oil can also be used to make scented candles, as it has a mild aroma that blends well with various fragrances.

Adhesives and Sealants

Castor oil is utilized in the manufacturing of adhesives and sealants due to its excellent adhesive properties and ability to provide a strong bond.

It is commonly used in the production of wood glues, construction adhesives, and sealants for its durability and long-lasting adhesive strength.

Industrial Coatings and Paints

Castor oil is an essential ingredient in the production of industrial coatings and paints due to its film-forming properties and ability to improve adhesion to various surfaces. It contributes to the durability, flexibility, and water resistance of coatings and paints, making them suitable for applications such as automotive coatings, marine coatings, and protective coatings.

Biofuel Production

Castor oil has gained attention as a potential feedstock for biofuel production. It possesses high viscosity and energy content, making it a promising renewable resource for biodiesel production. The cultivation of castor beans for biofuel can contribute to sustainable energy production and reduce dependence on fossil fuels.

Chapter 5: Precautions and Considerations

Precautions and ... network

Allergic Reactions and Sensitivities

Although rare, some individuals may have allergic reactions or sensitivities to castor oil. Before using castor oil topically, perform a patch test by applying a small amount to a small area of skin and observing for any adverse reactions such as redness, itching, or irritation.

If you experience any signs of an allergic reaction, discontinue use immediately and consult a healthcare professional.

Internal Use and Dosage

Internal use of castor oil should be done cautiously and under professional guidance. Castor oil has a laxative effect and can cause gastrointestinal discomfort if taken in excess or without proper dosage instructions. Consult a healthcare professional or follow recommended dosage guidelines if using castor oil internally for digestive issues.

Choosing High-Quality Castor Oil

- Ensure that you select high-quality, pure castor oil for optimal effectiveness and safety.

- Look for cold-pressed or organic castor oil options as these tend to retain more of the natural beneficial compounds.

- Check for reputable brands and read product labels to ensure you are purchasing a reliable and authentic product.

Proper Storage and Shelf Life

Store castor oil in a cool, dark place away from direct sunlight to maintain its potency and extend its shelf life. Castor oil has a relatively long shelf life, usually ranging from one to two years, but it is still advisable to check the expiration date and discard any expired products.

Avoid Contact with Eyes and Mucous Membranes

Keep castor oil away from direct contact with the eyes and mucous membranes, as it can cause irritation and discomfort. If accidental contact occurs, rinse the affected area thoroughly with water and seek medical attention if necessary.

Consult a Healthcare Professional

If you have any underlying health conditions, are pregnant o

breastfeeding, or are taking medications, it is advisable t

consult a healthcare professional before using castor oil. The

can provide personalized guidance and ensure that castor oil i

safe for your specific circumstances.

Chapter 6: Castor Oil Packs

In the realm of natural remedies and holistic wellness, few substances hold the mystique and healing potential of castor oil This chapter explores the age-old practice of using castor oil packs, a time-tested remedy that harnesses the power of this remarkable oil to promote healing, detoxification, and overall well-being.

Preparing Your Healing Elixir

The cornerstone of harnessing castor oil's power lies in the preparation of castor oil packs. Creating your healing elixir is simple and requires only a few essential ingredients:

1. **Castor Oil**: Opt for a high-quality, cold-pressed, and organic castor oil to ensure purity and effectiveness.

2. **Flannel or Wool Cloth**: Choose a piece of cloth large enough to cover the area you wish to treat. Flannel or wool works best due to their ability to absorb and hold the oil.

3. **Plastic Wrap or Bag**: To protect your bedding or clothing, you'll need plastic wrap or a plastic bag to cover the castor oil-soaked cloth.

4. **Hot Water Bottle or Heating Pad**: To enhance the absorption of the oil, you'll need a source of gentle heat.

The Art of Applying a Castor Oil Pack

1. **Preparation**: Lay out your materials and ensure you have a clean, quiet space for your treatment. It's best to do this before bedtime as you'll want to relax for an hour or two afterward.

2. **Fold and Soak**: Fold the cloth to an appropriate size, typically around 8x8 inches. Soak the cloth in castor oil until it's saturated but not dripping.

3. **Application**: Lie down comfortably and place the castor oil-soaked cloth on the targeted area. Common areas include the abdomen, liver, kidneys, or joints. Cover the cloth with plastic wrap or a plastic bag to prevent oil from seeping out.

4. **Heat and Relaxation**: Place the hot water bottle or heating pad over the plastic-covered cloth. The gentle heat helps the oil penetrate deeper into the skin and tissues. Now, take this time to relax. Read a book, meditate, or simply unwind.

5. **Duration**: Leave the pack in place for at least 30 minutes, but you can keep it on for several hours or even overnight if comfortable.

6. **Cleanse and Store**: Afterward, remove the castor oil pack and cleanse the area with warm water and mild soap. Store the cloth in a sealed container for future use. Note that you can reuse the same cloth multiple times; just re-soak it in castor oil before each application.

The Healing Benefits

Castor oil packs offer a wide range of potential benefits:

- **Detoxification**: They help stimulate lymphatic circulation and liver function, aiding the body in eliminating toxins and waste.

- **Pain Relief**: The anti-inflammatory properties of castor oil can provide relief from various types of pain, including menstrual cramps, joint pain, and muscle soreness.

- **Digestive Support**: Applying packs to the abdomen can improve digestion and relieve constipation.

- **Skin Health**: Castor oil is renowned for its ability to promote healthy skin, reduce inflammation, and combat acne.

- **Stress Reduction**: The relaxation induced during the treatment can reduce stress and promote a sense of well-being.

Incorporating castor oil packs into your holistic wellness routine can be a transformative experience. However, it's essential to consult with a healthcare professional before beginning any new treatment, especially if you have underlying health conditions or are pregnant.

In the journey to optimal health, castor oil packs serve as a gentle yet powerful ally, offering a holistic approach to healing and rejuvenation. So, prepare your castor oil pack, lay back, and let the ancient healing power of this elixir work its magic.

Chapter 7: Why do I love Castor Oil Packs? A Personal Journey

As I sit down to pen this chapter, I can't help but feel a profound

sense of gratitude for the remarkable healing journey that castor

oil packs have guided me on. This chapter is a personal account

of my deep-seated affection for these simple yet transformative

treatments and how they've played a pivotal role in addressing

various health issues in my life.

A Lifelong Quest for Wellness

My journey with holistic health and natural remedies began

many years ago. Frustrated with the limitations of conventional

medicine and its propensity for treating symptoms rather than

root causes, I embarked on a mission to explore alternative

approaches to healing. It was during this quest that I first

encountered castor oil packs.

Finding Relief for Chronic Pain

One of the most profound ways castor oil packs impacted my life was by offering relief from chronic pain. For years, I grappled with persistent joint pain, which often left me feeling defeated and exhausted. After hearing about the anti-inflammatory properties of castor oil, I decided to give it a try. Applying a castor oil pack to my sore joints became a nightly ritual. The soothing warmth and the gradual reduction in pain were nothing short of miraculous. Over time, my reliance on painkillers diminished, and I began to regain a sense of control over my life. It was my first taste of the healing power of castor oil, and I was hooked.

A Remedy for Digestive Woes

Digestive issues had also plagued me for years. Frequent bouts of bloating, indigestion, and constipation left me feeling perpetually uncomfortable. Desperate for relief, I explored various dietary changes and supplements, but it was the introduction of castor oil packs over my abdomen that truly made a difference.

The packs seemed to work in harmony with my body, promoting better digestion and regularity. The gentle massage effect, combined with the oil's anti-inflammatory properties, provided much-needed relief. My digestive system began to function more smoothly, and I was no longer a prisoner to my stomach troubles.

A Companion in Self-Care

Beyond their physical benefits, castor oil packs also became a cherished part of my self-care routine. The act of setting aside time for myself, lying down with a warm pack, and embracing relaxation offered a sanctuary in the midst of life's chaos. It became an opportunity to reconnect with my body, mind, and spirit.

As I closed my eyes during those sessions, I often found a sense of serenity and clarity that eluded me in the rush of daily life. The castor oil packs became a symbol of self-love and self-preservation, a reminder that nurturing oneself is not a luxury but a necessity.

Chapter 8: Castor Oil's Vision Quest

As I delved deeper into the world of castor oil and its incredible healing properties, my curiosity led me down a path I hadn't initially expected - the potential benefits of castor oil for vision improvement. What I uncovered not only surprised me but also brought into focus the remarkable potential of this ancient elixir.

My Personal Journey with Castor Oil and Vision

My journey into the world of castor oil and its impact on vision began with a simple curiosity about holistic remedies for eye health. Having worn glasses for most of my life and experiencing occasional discomfort and strain, I wondered if there was a natural solution that could offer some relief. That's when I stumbled upon stories of castor oil's potential to improve eyesight.

Armed with hope and a small bottle of castor oil, I embarked on an experiment. I started by applying a tiny drop of castor oil to each closed eyelid before bedtime, gently massaging it in with my fingertips. At first, the sensation was unusual, but it wasn't uncomfortable. I felt a soothing warmth and an immediate sense of relaxation. Over the course of several weeks, I adhered to this ritual diligently. To my surprise, I began noticing subtle changes. My eyes felt less fatigued at the end of long workdays, and I could read for longer periods without experiencing the usual strain. While my vision didn't miraculously return to perfect clarity, it was apparent that something positive was happening. Castor oil had subtly, but noticeably, improved my eye comfort and stamina.

The Eye Floater Mystery Solved

As I continued my exploration into castor oil's potential benefits for vision, I stumbled upon the success story from my dear friend Sarah. Sarah had been plagued by the presence of eye floaters for years. These tiny, shadowy specks drifting across her field of vision had been a source of constant frustration and anxiety. Traditional medicine had offered no solution, and she had resigned herself to live with this persistent nuisance.

Sarah's journey with castor oil began when I told her about its potential to dissolve and eliminate eye floaters. Skeptical but desperate for relief, she decided to give it a try. Using a clean dropper, she applied a single drop of castor oil to each eye every night before bed. Weeks turned into months, and Sarah noticed a gradual but undeniable improvement. The eye floaters that had plagued her for so long began to dissipate after two months of diligent use. The once-distorted clarity of her vision returned, and with each passing day, her eyes became more comfortable and her confidence in castor oil grew.

A Holistic Approach to Vision

My experience and Sarah's story are testaments to the potential benefits of castor oil for vision improvement. While it may not offer a magical solution, castor oil can undoubtedly contribute to eye comfort, reduced strain, and, in some cases, the alleviation of certain eye conditions.

But as with any holistic approach to health, it's essential to remember that results can vary from person to person. What worked for me and my friend might not work for everyone. Castor oil should be used as part of a comprehensive eye-care plan, alongside regular eye exams and consultation with healthcare professionals. In this journey through the world of astor oil, I've come to appreciate its multifaceted nature. From

ealing aches and pains to nurturing the skin, and now, gently

upporting vision, castor oil continues to amaze me with its

ersatility and potential to enhance well-being. It serves as a

eminder that the wisdom of ancient remedies still holds power

1 our modern world, waiting to be explored and appreciated

new.

A Journey of Discovery

My love for castor oil packs extends beyond their physical benefits. It's about the profound connection I've developed with this ancient remedy and the empowerment it has brought into my life. Through this journey, I've realized that true healing goes beyond the surface; it involves understanding and honoring the intricate interplay of the body, mind, and soul.

While my experiences with castor oil packs have been undeniably positive, it's essential to remember that every individual is unique. What works for one person may not work for another. It's crucial to approach holistic remedies with an open mind, seeking guidance from healthcare professionals when needed and listening to the wisdom of your own body.

In conclusion, castor oil packs have become more than just a healing tool for me; they are a symbol of empowerment, self-discovery, and holistic wellness. As you continue your own journey of exploration, I encourage you to remain open to the possibilities that lie ahead, for the path to wellness is as unique as the individual who walks it.

Chapter 8: Recapitulation

Congratulations! You have now completed your comprehensive journey into the world of castor oil. Throughout this guide, we have explored the remarkable properties, historical significance, and versatile applications of this nature's elixir. From health and beauty to industrial uses, castor oil has proven its worth as a powerful and multifaceted substance.

By embracing castor oil, you have unlocked the potential for enhancing your well-being, nurturing your skin and hair, supporting your health, and contributing to sustainable practices. This guide has provided you with insights into the science behind castor oil, its production methods, and its extensive range of applications. Armed with this knowledge, you can confidently incorporate castor oil into your daily life, benefiting from its exceptional qualities.

Remember, as you explore the possibilities of castor oil, it is essential to follow precautions and considerations to ensure your safety and maximize its effectiveness. Perform patch tests, consult healthcare professionals when needed, and choose high-quality products to optimize your experience.

Whether you are seeking natural remedies for skincare concerns, aiming to promote wellness, or exploring sustainable alternatives in various industries, castor oil offers a world of possibilities. Its remarkable versatility, combined with its rich history and proven benefits, make it a valuable resource for those seeking to harness the power of nature.

We hope this comprehensive guide has inspired you to explore and embrace the remarkable potential of castor oil. Now, armed with knowledge and understanding, it's time to embark on your own castor oil journey. Experiment, create, and experience the transformative effects of this incredible elixir.

Thank you for joining us on this exploration of castor oil. May it bring you health, beauty, and a deep connection to the wonders of nature. Embrace the power of castor oil and let it enrich your

life in countless ways.

Appendix: DIY Recipes and Remedies

n this appendix, we present a collection of simple and effective

do-it-yourself (DIY) recipes and remedies using castor oil.

These recipes allow you to harness the power of castor oil and

create your own natural remedies and beauty treatments.

Remember to perform a patch test before using any new recipe

and discontinue use if you experience any adverse reactions.

Moisturizing Castor Oil Face Mask

Ingredients:

- 1 tablespoon castor oil

- 1 tablespoon honey

- 1 tablespoon plain yogurt

Instructions:

1. In a small bowl, mix the castor oil, honey, and yogurt unti well combined.

2. Apply the mixture to your clean face, avoiding the eye area.

3. Leave the mask on for 15-20 minutes.

4. Rinse off with warm water and follow with your regular skincare routine.

5. Enjoy the nourishing and moisturizing benefits of this mask for soft, hydrated skin.

Strengthening Castor Oil Hair Serum

Ingredients:

- 2 tablespoons castor oil
- 1 tablespoon coconut oil
- 5 drops rosemary essential oil

Instructions:

1. In a small glass bottle, combine the castor oil, coconut oil and rosemary essential oil.
2. Shake well to mix the ingredients thoroughly.
3. Apply a few drops of the serum to your fingertips and massage it into your scalp.
4. Gently work the serum through your hair, focusing on the ends.
5. Leave the serum in overnight or for a few hours before shampooing and conditioning as usual.

6. Use regularly to nourish and strengthen your hair, promoting healthier growth.

Soothing Castor Oil Compress for Joint Pain

Ingredients:

- 2 tablespoons castor oil
- Soft, clean cloth or flannel
- Hot water bottle or heating pad

Instructions:

1. Pour the castor oil onto the center of the cloth or flannel.
2. Fold the cloth to enclose the castor oil, creating a compress.
3. Place the compress over the affected joint area.
4. Apply a hot water bottle or heating pad on top of the compress to provide gentle warmth.
5. Leave the compress in place for 30-60 minutes, allowing the heat and castor oil to penetrate.
6. Remove the compress and store it in a sealed container for reuse.

7. Repeat as needed to alleviate joint pain and promote relaxation.

Nourishing Castor Oil Lip Balm

Ingredients:

- 1 tablespoon castor oil

- 1 tablespoon beeswax pellets

- 1 tablespoon coconut oil

- Optional: a few drops of your favorite essential oi
  (e.g., peppermint, lavender)

Instructions:

1. In a double boiler or microwave-safe bowl, melt the casto
   oil, beeswax pellets, and coconut oil together.

2. Stir well until all ingredients are completely melted and
   combined.

3. If desired, add a few drops of your favorite essential oil fo
   fragrance and additional benefits.

4. Pour the mixture into lip balm containers or small jars.

5. Allow it to cool and solidify completely before using.

6. Apply the lip balm to moisturize and nourish your lips, leaving them soft and supple.

Revitalizing Castor Oil Eye Serum

Ingredients:

- 1 tablespoon castor oil

- 1 teaspoon vitamin E oil

- 3-4 drops rosehip oil

Instructions:

1. In a small glass bottle, combine the castor oil, vitamin E oil and rosehip oil.

2. Shake well to blend the ingredients thoroughly.

3. Apply a small amount of the serum to your clean fingertips.

4. Gently pat the serum around the delicate eye area, avoiding direct contact with the eyes.

5. Use this revitalizing eye serum nightly to hydrate the skin, reduce the appearance of fine lines, and improve the overall appearance of the eye area.

Castor Oil Hair Mask with Coconut Oil

Ingredients:

- 2 tablespoons of castor oil

- 1 tablespoon of coconut oil

Instructions:

1. In a small bowl, combine the castor oil and coconut oil.

2. Heat the mixture for a few seconds until it's warm but not too hot to touch.

3. Apply the warm oil mixture to your scalp and hair, massaging it in gently.

4. Cover your hair with a shower cap or a warm towel.

5. Leave the mask on for at least 30 minutes, or you can leave it overnight for better results.

6. Wash your hair thoroughly with a mild shampoo and conditioner.

Castor Oil and Aloe Vera Hair Serum

Ingredients:

- 2 tablespoons of castor oil

- 2 tablespoons of aloe vera gel

Instructions:

1. In a small bowl, mix the castor oil and aloe vera gel until you get a smooth, consistent mixture.

2. Apply this serum to your scalp and massage it in gently fo a few minutes.

3. Leave the serum on for 1-2 hours.

4. Rinse your hair thoroughly with a mild shampoo and conditioner.

Castor Oil and Egg Hair Mask

Ingredients:

2 tablespoons of castor oil

1 egg

1 tablespoon of honey (optional, for added moisture)

Instructions:

. In a bowl, whisk the egg until it's well-beaten.

. Add the castor oil and honey (if using) to the egg and mix

thoroughly.

. Apply this mixture to your hair and scalp, making sure to

cover all areas.

. Leave the mask on for about 30-45 minutes.

. Rinse your hair with cold water to prevent the egg from

cooking, then shampoo and condition as usual.

Castor Oil and Rosemary Oil Hair Growth Tonic

Ingredients:

- 2 tablespoons of castor oil

- 5-7 drops of rosemary essential oil

Instructions:

1. In a small glass bottle, combine the castor oil and rosemary essential oil.

2. Shake well to mix the oils thoroughly.

3. Before bedtime, apply a few drops of this mixture to your scalp and massage it in gently.

4. Leave it on overnight.

5. In the morning, wash your hair with a mild shampoo. These recipes can be used once or twice a week, depending on your preference and hair type. Keep in mind that consistency is key when using natural remedies like

castor oil for hair growth, and results may vary from

person to person. If you experience any irritation or

discomfort, discontinue use and consult a dermatologist or

healthcare professional.

Luxurious Whipped Shea Butter and Castor Oil Body Butter

Ingredients:

- 1/2 cup shea butter

- 1/4 cup coconut oil

- 1/4 cup castor oil

- 10-15 drops of your favorite essential oil (e.g., lavender, vanilla, or citrus for fragrance)

Instructions:

1. In a double boiler or microwave, melt the shea butter and coconut oil until they're completely liquid. Stir to combine.

2. Let the mixture cool for a few minutes, but it should still be in a liquid state.

3. Add the castor oil and essential oil of your choice to the mixture and stir to combine.

4. Place the mixture in the refrigerator for about 15-20 minutes or until it starts to set around the edges.

5. Using a hand mixer or stand mixer, whip the mixture on high speed for about 5-7 minutes or until it becomes light and fluffy.

6. Spoon the whipped body butter into a clean, airtight container.

Soothing Cocoa Butter and Castor Oil Body Butter

Ingredients:

- 1/2 cup cocoa butter

- 1/4 cup castor oil

- 1/4 cup sweet almond oil

- 10-15 drops of lavender or chamomile essential oil (for a soothing effect)

Instructions:

1. In a double boiler or microwave, melt the cocoa butter until it's completely liquid. Stir to combine.

2. Add the castor oil and sweet almond oil to the melted cocoa butter, and mix well.

3. Allow the mixture to cool slightly but not solidify.

4. Add your chosen essential oil and mix thoroughly.

5. Place the mixture in the refrigerator for about 15-20 minutes until it begins to solidify around the edges.

6. Using a hand mixer or stand mixer, whip the mixture until it becomes fluffy and resembles the texture of whipped cream.

7. Transfer the whipped body butter into a clean, airtight container.

To use these body butters, simply scoop out a small amount and apply it to your skin. The warmth of your skin will melt the butter, making it easy to spread. These body butters are excellent for dry skin and can be applied all over the body, especially after a shower or bath. Store them in a cool, dry place, and they should keep well for several months. Enjoy the luxurious, moisturizing benefits of these homemade body butters!

Basic Castor Oil Toothpaste

Ingredients:

- 4 tablespoons baking soda

- 2 tablespoons coconut oil

- 1 tablespoon castor oil

- 10 drops peppermint essential oil (for flavor and freshness

Instructions:

1. In a small mixing bowl, combine the baking soda, coconu

   oil, and castor oil.

2. Add the peppermint essential oil for flavor and mix well

   until you achieve a paste-like consistency.

3. Store your homemade toothpaste in an airtight container.

To use, simply dip your toothbrush into the paste or use a small

spoon to scoop a small amount onto your toothbrush. Brush

your teeth as you normally would. This toothpaste provides a

natural way to clean and freshen your breath.

Herbal Castor Oil Toothpaste

Ingredients:

- 3 tablespoons calcium carbonate powder (food grade)

- 2 tablespoons baking soda

- 1 tablespoon castor oil

- 10-15 drops tea tree essential oil (for its antibacterial properties)

- 5-7 drops peppermint essential oil (for flavor and freshness)

- Dried herbs (optional, for added herbal benefits; e.g., sage or thyme)

Instructions:

1. In a small mixing bowl, combine the calcium carbonate powder and baking soda.

2. Add the castor oil, tea tree essential oil, and peppermint essential oil to the dry mixture. Mix until you achieve a paste-like consistency.

3. If desired, add dried herbs for added herbal benefits and mix well.

4. Transfer your homemade herbal castor oil toothpaste into an airtight container.

Use this toothpaste just like you would any commercial toothpaste. The calcium carbonate helps to gently polish the teeth, while the castor oil and tea tree oil provide antibacterial properties. The peppermint oil adds a pleasant flavor and freshens breath.

Keep in mind that homemade toothpaste may not contain fluoride, so if you prefer fluoride in your toothpaste, consult your dentist for recommendations. Also, if you have any allergies or sensitivities to the ingredients used, consider alternative toothpaste options. Homemade toothpaste can be a fun and natural alternative, but it's important to maintain good oral hygiene and visit your dentist regularly for check-ups.

Castor Oil Nail and Cuticle Oil

Ingredients:

- 1 tablespoon castor oil

- 1 tablespoon sweet almond oil (or another carrier oil of your choice)

- 5-7 drops of lavender essential oil (optional, for a pleasant scent and added nail benefits)

Instructions:

1. In a small glass bottle, combine the castor oil and sweet almond oil.

2. If desired, add a few drops of lavender essential oil for fragrance and extra nail care benefits.

3. Seal the bottle and shake well to mix the oils thoroughly.

4. Apply a drop of the oil mixture to each nail and massage i

   gently into the nail and cuticle area.

5. Allow the oil to absorb for at least 15-20 minutes, or leave

   it on overnight for an intensive treatment.

6. For best results, use this nail and cuticle oil daily or as

   needed to strengthen and moisturize your nails.

Castor Oil Nail and Lemon Juice Soak

Ingredients:

- 1 tablespoon castor oil

- Juice of half a lemon

- A small bowl of warm water

Instructions:

1. In a small bowl, mix the castor oil and freshly squeezed lemon juice.

2. Fill another small bowl with warm water and soak your nails in it for about 5-10 minutes to soften them.

3. After soaking, pat your nails dry with a towel.

4. Apply the castor oil and lemon juice mixture to your nails and cuticles, massaging it in gently.

5. Leave the mixture on for about 15-20 minutes.

6. Rinse your nails with warm water and pat them dry.

The lemon juice in this recipe can help brighten and whiten you

nails, while the castor oil strengthens and moisturizes them.

Consistency is key when using these treatments. Regular

application can help improve the strength and overall health of

your nails over time. Keep in mind that nails grow slowly, so it

may take a few weeks or even months to see significant results.

Additionally, if you have any allergies or skin sensitivities,

perform a patch test before using any new nail treatments.

Sugar and Castor Oil Scrub

Ingredients:

- 1/4 cup brown sugar (or granulated sugar for a gentler scrub)

- 1 tablespoon castor oil

- 1-2 drops of your favorite essential oil (e.g., lavender, tea tree, or citrus)

Instructions:

1. In a small bowl, combine the sugar and castor oil.

2. Add a few drops of your chosen essential oil for fragrance and additional skin benefits. Mix well.

3. Use this mixture to gently scrub your face or body in circular motions, avoiding the eye area.

4. Rinse with warm water and pat your skin dry.

5. Follow with your regular moisturizer if needed.

This sugar and castor oil scrub can help remove dead skin cells, leaving your skin feeling soft and refreshed. The castor oil provides moisture, while the sugar acts as a natural exfoliant.

Castor Oil and Oatmeal Exfoliating Mask

Ingredients:

- 1 tablespoon castor oil

- 1 tablespoon finely ground oats (oat flour)

- 1-2 teaspoons plain yogurt (or honey for additional moisture)

Instructions:

1. In a small bowl, combine the castor oil, finely ground oats, and yogurt (or honey).

2. Mix the ingredients to create a thick paste.

3. Apply this paste to your clean, damp face and gently massage it in using circular motions.

4. Leave the mask on for about 10-15 minutes.

5. Rinse off the mask with warm water and pat your skin dry.

This exfoliating mask combines the exfoliating properties of oatmeal with the moisturizing and cleansing properties of castor oil. The yogurt or honey adds extra moisture and can help soothe the skin.

When using homemade exfoliants, it's essential to be gentle, especially on the face. Over-exfoliating can damage the skin, so limit exfoliation to 1-2 times a week or as needed for your skin type. Always perform a patch test before using any new skincare product to ensure you don't have any adverse reactions.

Relaxing Castor Oil Bath Soak

Ingredients:

- 1 cup Epsom salt

- 2 tablespoons castor oil

- 5-6 drops lavender essential oil

Instructions:

1. In a bowl, combine the Epsom salt, castor oil, and lavender essential oil.

2. Mix well until the ingredients are evenly distributed.

3. Add the mixture to a warm bath and stir to dissolve.

4. Soak in the bath for 20-30 minutes, allowing the castor oil and Epsom salt to relax your muscles and promote a sense of calm.

5. Rinse off with warm water after the bath.

Glossary

1. **Castor Oil:** A vegetable oil derived from the seeds of the castor bean plant (Ricinus communis). It is known for its various properties and wide range of applications.

2. **Ricinoleic Acid:** The primary fatty acid found in castor oil, responsible for its unique properties such as anti-inflammatory, antimicrobial, and analgesic effects.

3. **Viscosity:** The measure of a fluid's resistance to flow. Castor oil has a high viscosity, making it thick and sticky in consistency.

4. **Cold-Pressed Castor Oil:** Castor oil obtained through mechanical pressing of castor beans without the use of heat or chemical solvents. It is often considered a pure and unrefined form of castor oil.

5. **Refining:** The process of further purifying and processing castor oil to remove impurities, enhance clarity, and improve stability.

6. **Pharmaceutical Grade:** Castor oil that meets specific quality standards for use in pharmaceutical and medical applications.

7. **Industrial Grade:** Castor oil used in industrial applications such as lubricants, coatings, and plastics.

8. **Cosmetic Grade:** Castor oil that meets quality standards for use in cosmetic and personal care products.

9. **Organic Castor Oil:** Castor oil produced from castor beans cultivated using organic farming practices, free from synthetic fertilizers and pesticides.

10. **Emollient:** An ingredient that helps soften and soothe the skin, providing hydration and moisturization.

11. **Antimicrobial:** Having properties that help inhibit the growth of microorganisms such as bacteria and fungi.

12. **Anti-inflammatory:** Acting to reduce inflammation and alleviate associated symptoms such as redness, swelling, and discomfort.

13. **Laxative:** A substance that promotes bowel movements and alleviates constipation.

14. **Patch Test:** A small-scale test performed by applying a product to a small area of skin to check for any adverse reactions or allergies.

15. **Essential Oil:** A concentrated liquid containing volatile aroma compounds extracted from plants, often used for their therapeutic properties and fragrance.

16. **Biofuel:** A fuel derived from renewable biological resources, such as castor oil, that can be used as an alternative to conventional fossil fuels.

17. **Adhesion:** The ability of a substance to stick to a surface or create a bond.

18.   **Sustainability:** The practice of using resources in a way that meets present needs without compromising the ability of future generations to meet their needs.

Made in the USA
Las Vegas, NV
01 October 2023

78363637R00075